Also by Dr. Stenbeck

Available from the usual on-line source

Books
Healing Yourself -- The Holistic Approach
  [An introduction to Holistic Self-healing.]

Heal Yourself Right Now!
  [The Seven Priority Organ Levels for
  effective Nutritional/Holistic Treatment of
  all organs.]

The 22 Unique Body Types
  (for Health and Weight Loss)

Q & A to Identify Your Body Type (Booklet)
  [Individual Type booklets are also available

Booklets
(Step-by-step instructions on healing yourself)

  #1 Start Healing with Positive Thinking
  #2 Mastering Positive Feelings for Health!
  #3 Spiritual Balance and Your Healing

The Pargenic Body Type

Representing one of the 22 Body Types first described by Victor Rocine around 1900

The Burt Reynolds, Katey Segal Celebrity Body Type

For Kaye,
there at the beginning with Doc Severn,
and for Liberty,
continuing the holistic healing journey...

Disclaimer

The information in this book is for educational purposes only and is not a substitute for medication, diets, or other medical care. The diets do not treat diseases or medical conditions, and are an adjunct to your orthodox health care.

The author and publisher accept no responsibility for any misuse of the information within. If you have any physical problem, food allergy, emotional disorder, or disease, common sense dictates that you consult with a physician before changing your diet, taking nutritional supplements, or following the advice given here.

About the Author

Educated in New Zealand and in the U.S.A., Dr. Stenbeck attained B.Sc. (NZ), M.S., and D.C. degrees. His holistic healing methods have been profiled in magazines (Esquire, McLean's, Playgirl, the Atlanta Constitution), and on TV in the USA and in Canada. He was the main contributor to the Warner Book, _The Eye/Body Connection_ by Jessica Maxwell that focused on the holistic healing relationships between the iris structure and organ genetics.

In the 1970-80's he was elected Fellow, Royal Society of Health, London; Fellow, American Association of Chemists; Member, American Association of Clinical Chemists; and Affiliate, Royal Society of Medicine, London. He studied naturopathy and Body Types with Dr. Bernard Jensen and Dr. Clifford Severn, and has practiced in medical partnerships where patients received the joint benefits of medical and holistic healing.

He is a member of Self-Realization Fellowship. To receive advice on any health issue from a holistic viewpoint, or to receive help with your body type, see his web site: *DrStenbeck.net*

———

Contents

* * *

The Pargenic Body Type and Food Guide   1

The 22 Body Types:
Celebrity Examples

This Booklet contains the Pargenic type. See <u>*The 22 Unique Body Types*</u> *for all type descript- ions.]*

Thin Types

Atrophic	*Woody Allen / Audrey Hepburn Stan Laurel / Calista Flockheart*
Exesthesic	*Cher / Sarah Jessica Parker (Female type only)*
Marasmic	*President Obama / Princess Diana James Stewart / Kate Blanchard*
Neurogenic	*J.K. Simmons / Joan Rivers Jon Cryer / Marin Hinle*
Pathoferic	*(No celebrity males) Blythe Danner / Gwyneth Paltrow*
Sillevitic	*David Bowie / Shirley MacLaine Rod Stewart / Carol Channing*

Muscle Types

Calciferic	*Michael Jordan / Angelica Huston* *Abraham Lincoln / Grace Jones*
Carbogenic	*George Clooney / Lady Gaga* *Pres. G. Bush, Jr. / Meg Ryan*
Desmogenic	*Marlon Brando / Loni Anderson* *Daniel Craig / Tina Turner*
Eldic	*Ross Perot / Hillary Clinton* *Peter Falk / Sigourney Weaver*
Medeic	*Gary Oldman / Madonna* *John Hurt / Marlene Deitrich*
Myogenic	*Pres. Bill Clinton / Sharon Stone* *Pres. John Kennedy / Julia Roberts*
Nervimotive	*Frank Sinatra / Elizabeth Taylor* *Mark Wahlberg / Natalie Wood*
Nitropheric	*Ben Affleck / Ava Gardner* *Kirk Douglas / Kate Winslet*
Pallinomic	*Pres. Donald Trump /* *Attorney General Janet Reno* *Bill O'Reilly (Fox) / Jane Russell*

Fat Types

Barotic   *Robin Williams / 'Mrs. Doubtfire'*
              Elton John / William Conrad

Carboferic   *Bill Murray / Roseanne*
              Billy Gardell / Melissa McCarthy

Hydripheric   *John Goodman / Shelly Winters*
              Wayne Knight / Jennifer Holliday

Isogenic   *Einstein / Oprah Winfrey*
              Phillip S .Hoffman / Queen Victoria

Lipopheric   *Rush Limbaugh / Rosie O'Donnell*
              Chris Christie / Camryn Manheim

Oxypheric   *Winston Churchill / Orsen Welles*
              Ella Fitzgerald / Gerry Spence

Pargenic   *Burt Reynolds / Katey Segal*
              Ron Perlman / Kirstey Alley

Succinct Quote on Human Types

From Victor Rocine, who first described discrete body types around 1900.

"A type is an order of people that differentiates and distinguishes itself by a general and similar form, brain-formation, chemistry, structure, build, immunity, tendencies, predisposition, resemblance, skin-pigment, and type characteristics based on observation and analogy.

"Or, in other words, people of a given type are similar physically and like-minded as if they were brothers and sisters—that is what type means.

"Everything in nature is made according to plan. Man only discovers that plan and gives it a name. The zoologist has not made the animals—he has only described the plan adopted by the wonderful Creator, and named the classes, sub-classes, etc.

"How important type research will be to humanity, time alone will make known."

———

Prologue

The esteemed scientist J. J. Berzelius, discoverer of several chemical elements, inspired Victor Rocine to research body types and to investigate the correlation between types and their diseases. Around 1890-1910, Rocine privately published his original findings on the mineral basis of different body types, and this present book exists because of his brilliant insights.

For many years, I studied with Dr. Clifford Severn who had been a personal student of Victor Rocine on body types, naturopathy, herbology, iris analysis, diet, and nutritional healing methods. He had a successful career as a lecturer and healer, and was one of those rare athletes with complete muscle control over his body. I saw him under a spotlight at 85 years of age, contracting and rippling every individual muscle in his perfectly developed body. Field-Marshal Jan Smuts, the WWII South African Prime Minister, devoted a full chapter of his autobiography to how Severn's healing methods had saved his life. In the 1950's, *Life* magazine did a four-page spread on Severn and his family. Fame he had.

Another Rocine student I studied with, Dr. Bernard Jensen wrote of Rocine's body type research and nutritional methods in his privately published, *The Chemistry of Man*.

This book is deeply rooted in Rocine's original work, and with that of Herbert Shelton, M.D., Ph.D. (at Harvard University in the 1930's). I integrated their research with newer dietary and nervous system data along with celebrity examples of each type, hopefully, making this material easier to digest and more entertaining for the reader.

Gayelord Hauser, another Rocine student I knew, was a celebrated health book author. He wrote a popular book on Rocine's types in the 1940's, *Types and Temperaments;* reputedly, he also introduced yogurt to the western world.

This book exists because of Rocine's creative brilliance and original discoveries in natural healing.

▶ *Rocine: "The soul creates the body type."*

Rocine taught that the soul chooses a body type and brain to live in, thus presenting different experiences and life lessons to master. Why were *you* born the way you are?

That is something to think about, especially if it is true! What would your soul purpose be to live in a particular body type. I provide some thoughts on this issue in each type description and try to assess from my experience with your type the particular lessons of life presented therein.

Rocine was as brilliant in his way as an Abraham Lincoln, Michael Jordan, Michael Phelps, Tony Robbins, or a Daniel Day Lewis—all *calciferic* types—rare, leaders, innovative, brilliant, and highly intelligent in their different fields of endeavor.

Celebrity examples exist for most types, not a duplicate of you, but someone who has your essence in their body-mind individuality. Knowing your type allows you to become a better you!

The celebrity examples provide further help in identifying your body type.

▶ *Rocine's classic findings, the backbone of this book, are integrated with Sheldon's research and with other dietary and food issues including mental, emotional, and spiritual attributes,*

Many people take nutritional supplements and try different diets without a doctor's advice. If this is your choice, use common sense, listen to body responses, and discontinue any allergic reactions to foods or nutritional substances.

———

The Pargenic
Body Type

"You may also have a physical or psychological feature not representative of your type such as height, weight, appearance, talent, weakness, strength, etc., due to biochemical errors, environmental influences, racial or cultural differences, and congenital or genetic issues. Nevertheless, the type identification of the average person is usually clear."

—*Victor Rocine*

1

Pargenic Type Celebrity Examples

*If you think this is your type, be sure to look at **<u>on-line photographs</u>** of these examples. Look for general similarities to yourself. Note that sub-types cause the differences in appearance between members of the same type.*

————

POLITICS

> President Richard Nixon
> King Farouk (Egypt)
> Saddam Hussein (Iraq)
> General Noriega (Panama)
> Senator Al Frankin
> Senator Joe McCarthy

JUDICIARY

> Supreme Court Justice Thurgood Marshall

NOTABLE

> Eleanor Roosevelt

FILM

Ron Perlman	Jerry Lewis
Sean Connery	Burt Reynolds
Matt Damon	Karl Malden
Powers Boothe	Paul Schofield
Ed Begley Sr.	Lee J. Cobb
Jose Ferrer	Doug McClure
Raul Julia	Paul Soverino
Jaime Farr	Mandy Patinkin
Jack Palance	Robert Davi

Martin Clunes (BBC)
Arnold Swartzenegger
Francis Ford Coppola

Hillary Swank	Phoebe Cates
Karen Black	Katey Segal
Kirstie Alley	Torrey Spelling
Geena Davis	

Talia Shire ("Rocky")
Sofia Copppola

WORLD CHESS CHAMPION

Magnus Carlsen (the highest ranked chess
player of all time)

TV/COMEDY

Don Rickles	Red Fox
Gary Shandling	Joe Piscopo
John Schuck (TV)	Ross Hunter (TV)

David Letterman   Robert Kline

VOICE/MUSIC

Mel Torme   Wayne Newton
Luciano Pavarotti
Herb Jeffries (Duke Ellington vocalist)
Amy Winehouse

SPORTS

Roger Federer   Pete Sampras

Gore Vidal   Salaman Rushdie
Stephen King
Andrew Weil, M.D. (esteemed holistic
physician)

HISTORY

Oscar Wilde

OTHER

Monica Lewinski

[Note: I personally knew eight of the above celebrities, and many in everyday life, which contributed to my understanding of the type.]

You already know something about this type from their public persona and appearance, whether from seeing them yourself or from the celebrity examples. Blend such insights with the type descriptions and the types of your family and friends to discern their presence in your midst!

Read through the types, and if still confused see the *Appendix* for the personal type identification request from my website: *DrStenbeck.net*

———

▶ *The type questionnaire pinpoints the major features of that type: if the celebrity examples are unhelpful, you may be an unusual variant (in which case ignore the celebrity issue and give yourself 7 points on Question 1).*

———

Pargenic Type Questionnaire

These questions describe the generic type, and not specifically you! If any question ever applied to you, then choose the True answer!

For Question 1 only:

A = True	*B = Maybe*	*C = Untrue*
15 points	*7 points*	*1 point*

1. Physically identify with celebrity example _____

Then...

A = True	*B = Maybe*	*C = Untrue*
5 points	*3 points*	*1 point*

---

2. Height is close to:
   Males: 5'8-6'5   Females: 5'6-6'0   _____
3. Usual weight is close to:
   Males: 160-300+ Females: 150-300+   _____
4. Body medium-sized when young, but
   may be fat or obese later in life   _____
5. Muscles large, medium strength; have
   athletic potential   _____
6. Highly intelligent, many intellectuals   _____
7. Hard working, industrious, honest   _____
8. Upper arms fat and fleshy (moreso
   in females)   _____
9. Shoulders fleshy and broad   _____
10. Able to influence others   _____

11. Sensuous and seductive tendency _____
12. May crave adulation _____
13. Some are conceited and haughty _____
14. Some have unpolished manners _____
15. Head often large, bony, irregular, vase-shaped, with a large upper-forehead and base of the head _____
16. Jet-black hair (some brown shades), thinning, slight balding usually starts about age 30-40; hair oily in some _____
17. Brown, dark eyes usual; eyebrows, eyelashes stiff, sparse _____
18. Large fleshy nose _____
19. Some have pock-marked skin or acne-scars _____
20. A heavy protruding lower jaw; some have double chins _____
21. Upper lip normal; lower lip loose, thicker, blue-red _____
22. Usually irregular teeth, white or yellowing, fragile _____
23. Skin irregular, lumpy, scarred, flaky, oily, may be unhealthy _____
24. Chest broad and deep; bust is moderate or larger _____
25. A strong fatty neck is typical _____
26. Back large and broad; large gluteals _____
27. May be sarcastic _____
28. Usually large broad hips, abdomen; waist large and fatty _____
29. Gestures may be awkward, ungainly _____
30. Behaviors carefully considered _____

31. Cautious, mistrusting, proud   _____
32. Mind is slow, ponderous, and
    powerful once aroused   _____
33. Learn more from life than from books _____
34. Great reasoning power (many lawyers) _____
35. Do not please or appease anyone   _____
36. Tend to be caustic, argumentative   _____
37. Willpower very strong   _____
38. May be conceited, absent-minded   _____
39. Brave and daring   _____
40. Some are sociopathic or antisocial   _____
41. May have covert, clandestine interests _____
42. May dwell on conspiracy theories   _____
43. Some have manic-depression or other
    disorders history(and need medication) _____
44. A few are immoral   _____
45. Many have intuitive powers   _____
46. Have a disobedient nature   _____
47. Full of hates, fears, delusions   _____
48. May believe are a law unto yourself _____
49. May sulk or be sullen   _____
50. May live with disorder; being tidy
     is not a priority   _____
51. Mostly sensuous, seductive (sexually
    intense when young)   _____
52. Expression is resentful, cautious   _____
53. Dogmatic: expect to be heard and
    obeyed   _____
54. Easily depressed or moody   _____
55. Some have unpolished manners,
    others are elegant   _____
56. Mind is slow, ponderous, powerful   _____

57. Complain about own inadequacies _____
58. Dogmatic, often controlling _____
59. Talents in writing, acting, performing _____
60. Muscle building is effective _____
61. Have abilities in mental work _____
62. May be awkward, unsophisticated _____
63. Are untrusting, proud, selfish,
    dogmatic, controlling _____
64. Some are prone to drugs, sex, sugar,
    or alcohol addiction _____
65. High self-confidence and self-image _____

Scoring

For question #1:

A response: give 15 points   = _____
B response: give 7 points   = _____
C response: give 1 points   = _____

For questions #2—65:

A response: give 5 points   = _____
B response: give 3 points   = _____
C response: give 1 point   = _____

Total of the above points   = _____

Interpretation

149—300: PROBABLY Pargenic type

75—148: POSSIBLY Pargenic type

<75: NOT Pargenic type

The Pargenic Type

Rocine: "Pargenic means 'incorrect production.' You utilize more food <u>calcium, carbon, phosphorus and sulfur</u> than other types. Your intellectual power may be brilliant and unsurpassed."
[Quite a compliment from Rocine, about your powerful brain.]

———

You are slender during childhood. By age 20 the males are medium-sized, some larger, and the females may be slender into their 30's. By middle age both sexes often hold extra fat, although some of you remain medium-sized throughout life by right eating and exercising, or by having a lean sub-type.

The females are typically charismatic, plain or pretty, and sometimes lovely or beautiful as in actors Katey Sagal, Sofia Coppola, Kirstey Alley, Phoebe Cates, and Karen Black. Even with Arnold Schwarzenegger and Burt Reynolds, one can see there is a fat component to the body. Stockier examples are Frances Ford Coppola, Doug McClure, and Karl Malden.

The strong calcium component provides for strong bones and brain power, the carbon gives a flesh-forming tendency, and the phosphorus portends a nervous nature.

Some of the men are "heart-throbs" and Burt Reynolds was the most popular male star in the world for a decade. I know several men who are plain or ruggedly handsome with their olive skin and natural jet-black or silver-gray hair. Many everyday examples may be plain looking (depending on the sub-type). You show the full spectrum of appearance from plain to radiant beauty, and from being medium-sized to heavy.

▶ *Rocine: "Pargenic refers to a blemished genetic blueprint resulting in slight to marked deviations from normal—either physical or mental." [This may be so slight as to be unrecognizable and unnoticeable, or sometimes it reflects a minor genetic defect.]*

You are not refined or aristocratic like the *oxypheric.* Some of you may be difficult to love or live with. Of course, most of you are evolved examples with no negative traits.

———

Physical Similarity to Other Types

A. If medium-sized, you may be confused with -

The medium-sized *carbogenic* type (Alec Baldwin, Bernadette Peters), looks similar to the *pargenic,* but is more attractive and approachable. The *nervimotive* type (Richard Gere, Natalie Wood) is shapely, attractive, pleasant, sociable, and rarely fat.

B. If fat, you may be confused with -

The *carboferic* type (John Candy, Roseanne Barr) is somewhat similar, and may be more attractive and approachable.

––––––

Average Height and Weight

Males: 5'8--6'5 160--300+ pounds
Females: 5'6--6'0 150--300+ pounds

––––––

Pargenic Type Description

The type description represents how you appear in everyday society. You may have a sub-type that alters parts of this description.

Think of the celebrity examples as you read the descriptions. You may appear medium-sized when dressed, but when undressed your fleshiness or vulnerability to holding fat shows. When healthy, you look vibrant and youthful. In ill-health, you may have a bloated appearance.

Head — Your head is large, bony, sometimes irregular or vase-shaped, and heavy in the base; the central-forehead is notably large.

Hair — After age 30-40, many males have a thinning and balding tendency from the forehead backwards; in others, the hair may be unmanageable and oily.

▶ *Your hair is often beautiful and jet black (some brown) when young adults. Jet-black hair is present in the pargenic and nervimotive types (and when these types are present as a sub-type).*

Eyes — Brown or dark eyes are typical; the eyebrows and eyelashes are either stiff and disorderly, or sparse and lacking. Granular deposits may occur in the eyelids.

Ears — You tend to have irregularly-shaped and sized ears.

Nose — A larger nose with a shiny tip is common.

Face — If unhealthy, your face may be greasy, pock-marked or acne-scarred from childhood; the *desmogenic and medeic* types may also have this feature. A heavy protruding lower jaw is common. More rarely, if you have mastered your appetite for fatty and rich foods you have less fat in your face and body.

Mouth, Lips and Voice — The upper lip is usually normal-sized; the lower lip is often loose, and thick with blue-red coloring. When you speak one hears dogma: you expect to be heard and obeyed, your voice may be coarse, low-pitched, or strident.

Teeth — Your teeth are usually irregular, white or yellowing, and fragile with aging.

Skin — Your skin may be irregular, lumpy, scarred, or unhealthy with darkish tints (you need a nutrition doctor). Acne is common in childhood, and may persist throughout life with the males being particularly vulnerable to scarring.

▶*I have seen this skin condition many times: your skin may be unhealthy: the pores release waste-acids and local infection occurs in the skin. The skin may be healthy with a healthy diet.*

Neck — A thick, strong and oily neck is typical (unless healthy). You commonly develop a double chin.

Muscles — Your muscles are large and moderately strong, but you do not have great strength. Arnold Swartzenegger won awards for body development, not for muscle strength, but he probably has great strength due to a *desmogenic or pallinomic* sub-type.

Many of you are attracted to body building. You are able to build muscular bodies and look like the strongest men in the world—but usually you are not. I think Arnold would agree that if he stopped working out and eating right, fat would quickly take the place of his muscle definition; but you are strong and impressive looking!

In school, you are strong with great brain-body coordination; you find your way into wrestling, boxing, or football, and sports like tennis, where you have become world champions (Federer, Sampras).

Chest — The chest is broad and deep; the bust is moderate in size, sometimes large.

Back and Shoulders — The back and shoulders are large and broad in the lower region.

Hips and Abdomen — Large broad hips and abdomen are typical; your waist is heavy, large and fatty.

Arms and Legs — Your upper arms hold fat, the thighs are thick, and the ankles weak. Your gestures may be ungainly.

Joints — The bones and joints are weak and achy.

———

Pargenic Personality Traits

If you are this type many, but not all, of the following characteristics are present—you may have overcome or moderated the negatives, but recognize that you once had several of them.

You may have any of the following traits.

- Are highly assertive and social
- High self-confidence and self-image
- Are intelligent, rational, clever, or brilliant
- Are strong in autonomy and independence
- The mind is slow, ponderous and powerful

- Moaning or snoring during sleep is common
- Learn more from life than from books and school
- Have few close friends, but may know many people
- Strong willpower; don't try to please or appease others
- Are proud, cautious, grave, mistrusting, brave, and daring
- All behaviors are carefully considered before taking action
- Have great reasoning power (many lawyers and intellectuals)
- Your rational brain and intellect is strong, making faith and trust in God a difficult proposition.

▶ *I have known you to keep extensive dream records: some long enough to be screenplays!*

Potential Challenges

You may have evolved from or not experienced these general challenges, so don't dwell on them. While a few show these negative characteristics, most of you are normal, socially responsible people:

▶ *Rocine: "You usually appear unhappy, pessimistic, sensuous, distrustful, and cautious. You might say you are happy, but your family knows the truth. You become happy after developing a God relationship."*

- You tend to be dogmatic in speech
- May sulk and be silent for long periods
- May feel like you are a law unto yourself
- Usually make no effort to be liked by others
- May appear cold, strange, secretive, mysterious
- Psychologists may find you have strange beliefs
- Many appear unhappy and distrusting of others
- May be caustic, critical, bitter, and argumentative
- May be tempted and become pot, cocaine, and alcohol addicts
- Some are highly aggressive or destructive (and need medication)
- Rocine: "Some are selfish, uncultured, intrusive, and contrary."

▶ *Rocine was quite critical about this type. One hundred years later, I find his comments NOT to be true in the Western world, and for that reason I have minimized his negative commentary.*

―――――

Pargenic Stress Management

You have strong *mental* stress prevention giving you good resistance to internalizing this stress into your stomach, adrenals, and immune system. *Emotional* stress prevention is vulnerable, and any of the above challenges may need help. *[If needing help managing these stresses, see my prior books.]*

―――――

Love

You are attracted to types who are sensual and mentally strong.

―――――

Talents and Vocations

Abilities — *Mental work, managers, politicians, government, professionals*

You make superb criminal lawyers and are right for any work requiring brainpower like law, banking, and commerce.

► *I have known or observed you as: managers, actors, authors, lawyers (many), singers, writers, salesmen, doctors, scientists—and as homeless persons.*

The type information cannot predict your future, but you are capable of bringing a creative excellence or brilliance to whatever you do in life.

Inabilities — *Menial work*

Physical labor is contraindicated—you need mental or creative work.

Health Problems

When sick you commonly experience health problems or diseases in any of the following organs and tissues:

Lungs — Are weak and vulnerable to bronchitis and disease.

Lymphatic System — Toxins easily overburden your lymph system.

Skin — Acne, pustules, boils, etc., are common in childhood.

Digestive System — Often produces gas, constipation, and low back pain.

Liver — The liver is easily toxic and damaged by alcohol, drugs, etc.

Psychiatric Disorders — Some of you may be sociopathic, and require (Lithium, Prozac, etc.)

Pargenic Acid/Alkaline Factor

For your health and healing, your nervous system genetics require a specific ratio of acid to alkaline foods. You are born with **intermediate** dominance (between *para-sympathetic* and *sympathetic*), and need *balanced* acid and alkaline-ash food intake. (Ash refers to the minerals left in your body after metabolizing foods.) You may indulge in both food classes. Construct this approximate ratio of food selections:

> *But, for your healing, if in ill health or after about age 40-45, you need to aim for this approximate ratio of food selections:*
> *70% Fruits, salads, vegetables*
> *30% Proteins, carbohydrates*

▶*Approximate your food ratios. On any particular day, it does not matter if one meal is mostly alkaline and another mostly acid—just try to balance it out for the day! If you make a mistake, try again tomorrow. It is a subjective call that you make; what is done over time makes the difference to your health.*

———

The Pargenic Spiritual Factor

Skip this paragraph if uninterested in a philosophical perspective on your type!

▶ *Rocine: "The soul chooses the body type."*

If as souls, we choose the brain and body type to spend a lifetime in, it could be to learn certain spiritual lessons related to perfecting ourselves, and our humanity, in God's eyes. What lessons does the type bring you? Only you can really decide what those lessons are.

You know your weaknesses, faults, and behaviors towards others. You know things about yourself that Victor Rocine could never get from his research subjects when he first wrote about types. So search your mind for the answers. Each discrete type has challenges of life lessons, spiritual goals, etc., and some of yours may be:

Faith — Having a spiritual life is paramount to your happiness, but some of you have difficulty believing in a God. You benefit greatly with religion in your life.

Sexual Intensity or Addiction — Therapy is often helpful.

Excessively Intellectual — Humility is required in spite of your brilliance.

Stubborn and Disobedient — Learn flexibility, and conform with society.

Crave Admiration and Adulation — Share credit with others!

Arrogance — Many of you have egocentric and arrogance problems that moderate with spiritual growth.

———

A Pargenic Story...

Ursula, age 34, 5'7, 166 pounds, had jet-black hair, pale skin, and carried her weight well: she was shapely, but heavy. She complained about difficulty in losing weight and with overcoming depression. Prior examinations had ruled out any medical problems.

Her dietary evaluation showed excessive intake of carbon foods: sugars, fats, carbohydrates, starches, grains, and breads; she also ate excessive calcium and phosphorus foods: kelp, Swiss and cheddar cheese, turnip greens, almonds, brewer's yeast, parsley, corn tortillas.

Ursula showed deficits in her important type minerals of chloride and fluoride, and needed to eat brie, Roquefort and Swiss cheese, coconut, salt water fish, ham, raw cabbage, cod liver oil, and garlic. After making the dietary changes and releasing some emotional issues, her depressions lifted and she soon started losing weight.

———

Pargenic Type
Mineral Food Needs

Apply this mineral data to the diet following the Fat type descriptions.

Excessive Foods:

- *Calcium*
- *Carbon (simple carbohydrates)*
- *Sodium (salted, junk foods)*
- *Sulfur*
- *Nitrogen (beef)*

Deficient Foods:

- *Phosphorus*
- *Potassium*
- *Iron*
- *Sodium, Chloride (unsalted)*
- *Nitrogen (non-beef, vegetable)*

These deficient minerals are common deficiencies in your type, and predispose you to ill-health.
If ill, be sure to use these lists with your <u>daily</u> food intake. If not ill, eat from the food lists 3-4 days <u>weekly</u> for health maintenance.
All food lists are in descending order of concentration and value to you, choose servings of foods in the upper half of each list first!
One serving is ½ cup.

Pargenic Excessive Foods -

Calcium is excessive in your tissues. It is highly concentrated in your bones, joints, muscles, nerves, heart, teeth, and gums; if you have an illness or disease in any of these tissues avoiding calcium foods and supplements may be a significant healing factor.

Carbon, excessive in your type and in all fat or obese people, is found in every cell of your body as the basis of life. Minimize it.

Sodium from salted junk foods is excessive in your tissues. To preserve your health and weight control you should avoid junk foods and fulfill your sodium needs from the food list (without using the salt shaker).

Sulfur from raw or cooked foods is contraindicated.

Nitrogen from red meat is excessive in your diet (if eaten more than once weekly) causing excess waste acid accumulation and illnesses; eat poultry, fish and eggs no more than 3-4 days weekly, with vegetarian proteins like legumes (peas, beans), seeds, nuts, pasta on the other days.

———

Deficient Foods -

In illness or disease, it is important to correct these deficiencies.

Phosphorus, deficient in your tissues, is needed because of intense nervous system activity and brain exhaustion. You are always thinking, planning, and worrying about everything in your life, especially your health.

Potassium is deficient in your type. It is a dominant element in your tissues and is vital to your muscle, heart, and brain health. If diseased, taking potassium foods and supplements may be a significant healing factor.

Iron is often deficient in your tissues, causing anemia with fatigue, pallor, headaches, shortness of breath, and dizziness.

Sodium and chloride from non-salted foods is deficient in your type and is a key to removing water–weight.

Nitrogen from vegetable proteins is deficient (see above notes).

———

Minimize

Excessive Foods

Calcium: 0-2 servings/<u>week</u>

Kelp, Swiss and cheddar cheese, dulse, greens (collard, turnip, dandelion, beet), almonds, parsley, Brazil nuts, watercress, celery, goat milk, tofu, dried figs, buttermilk, yogurt, wheat bran, whole milk, ripe olives, broccoli, cottage cheese.

Carbon: 0-1 servings/week

Sugars, fats, carbohydrates, pasta, grains, breads, sweet fruits, alcohol, breads, butter, chocolate, cookies, pies, etc., all white sugar foods, honey.

Sodium (salted, junk): 0-1 servings/week

Salt, all fast foods, packaged foods, canned and frozen foods, preserved meats (cured, smoked, canned), sauces (soy, barbecue, catsup, etc.), dill pickles, sauerkraut, bouillon cubes, peanut butter, potato chips, etc., salted nuts, crackers, canned or packaged soups, processed cheeses, commercial salad dressings.

Note: If you must eat anything on the above lists, keep it down to ½ cup weekly!

Minimize…

Sulfur: *0-1 servings/week*

Cabbage, onions, cauliflower, garlic, Brussels sprouts, turnips, mustard greens, rutabagas, spinach, beans, carrots, horseradish. turnips, beans, horseradish, shrimp.

Nitrogen: *0-1 times weekly*

Beef, red meats

Eat

Deficient Foods

Phosphorus: *1-2 servings/day*

Soda water, Brewer's yeast, seeds (pumpkin, squash, sunflower, sesame), pinto beans, nuts (peanuts, walnuts, cashews, pecans), rye, beef-liver, scallops, wheat, barley, oats, eggs, lentils, garlic, crab, lamb, mushrooms.

Potassium, Iron: *1-2 servings/day*

Blackstrap molasses, rice, raisins, dark green leafy vegetables, dried prunes, yams, Swiss chard, parsnips, halibut, non-wheat whole grains, liver, organ meats, dried fruits, shellfish broths.

Eat...

Sodium, Chloride: *1-2 servings/day*

Scallops, lobster, gizzard, celery (and juice), raw cabbage and cauliflower, olives, gizzard, lentils, cheese (brie, Roquefort, cottage), sprouts, lobster, spinach, chicken, Swiss chard, beets and greens, salt water fish, lamb, turkey, pistachio, okra.

Nitrogen (non-beef, vegetable):

Legumes, peas, beans, black-eyed peas, pasta, spirulina, soybean products (tofu) — as desired

Eggs, poultry, fish: 3-5 times weekly

Note: Eat any healthy foods you desire, but be sure to include type foods in your daily choices.

Note: Eat any other healthy foods you desire, but be sure to include the type food suggestions in your daily choices.

Pargenic Nutritional Supplements

[Take all supplements with food.]

- **Multi-Vitamins** — *2 capsules/day*

- **Potassium** — *Take 99 mg/day*

- **Do not take Calcium or Multi-Minerals** —

  You already have excessive calcium in your body. (Exception: if highly stressed, menopausal, on estrogen, or osteoporotic)

- **Iron** — *25 mg/day with food (females)*

- **Herbs** —

  Brain detox – Chamomile or White Oak Organ detox – Fo-ti or Elderberry Leaf (Take one capsule, twice daily for one month; then one, three times weekly.)

- **Lecithin** — *1,300 mg/three times weekly*

  Note: Be sure to take these supplements if you have ill-health. If you are in good health, take them at least 3-4 times/week.

Note. The above recommendations are for the generic type. Additionally, you may need from a holistic healer or nutritionist something more specific for your individuality.

Important Pargenic Health Concerns

Your nervous system genetics require a *semi-vegetarian* Food Guide for health. In addition to taking the type minerals, it is essential that you limit red meat, fat, sugar, and alcohol intake.

PARGENIC FOOD GUIDE

Aim for -

70% Fruits, Salads, Vegetables
30% Proteins, Carbohydrates
and
70% Cooked foods
30% Raw food diet
Rocine: "Minimize red meats, fatty foods, cold drinks and starches and spices."

Minimize sulfur vegetables.
Take the recommended supplements.

Pargenic Weight Loss

Your body absorbs excessive fat from an early age, and you have great difficulty in losing it. Give yourself permission to exercise! It is essential for your fat burning. Follow theses these instructions and you will make good progress.

- *Drink* warm or hot citrus juices and clam or shellfish broths before choosing water!
- *Avoid* carbon, junk sodium, and cooked sulfur foods (see list)
- *Protein* drink in citrus juice daily, about 25-30 grams
- *Eat* your body type deficient mineral foods daily
- *Follow* your *Pargenic Guide (as above)*
- *Exercise*: your body type requires moderate to intense daily exercise (like walking or swimming)
- *Simple sugars*: stop all white table sugar and high-fructose corn syrup and drinks containing these sugars
- *If hypoglycemic* (low blood sugar, fatigue, depression, etc.), which stops fat loss and usually initiates more fat production, it is vital to deal with this problem: take *pantothenic acid,* 500 mg/twice daily with food (see my earlier books to resolve this problem)
- *Calories:* As with any dietary approach, calories in,- must be *less than* calories out! Most markets sell a calorie booklet; make notes of your daily intake, and in most

instances keep it under about 1500-1800 calories/day

———

Summary

You may think that the medium-sized *isogenic and pargenic* males are muscle types—and they do have strong muscles—study them and you will soon discern the differences.

———

Fat Types
General Food Guide

---

*(An Intermediate Guide between
Carnivores and Vegetarians)*

Important Note

———

The Food Guide addresses the <u>Acid-Alkaline</u> aspect of your food intake, along with the <u>Type Mineral</u> factor presented throughout this book. It does <u>not</u> necessarily address calories or other dietary factors that may be pertinent to your personal health needs whether medical or appropriate for some other dietary need. So use your common sense and just include the factors described here with whatever healthy dietary choices you usually make.

For other nutrient information, consult with nutritional books or with holistic nutritional doctors. In this regard, I particularly recommend the advice of Andrew Weil, M.D.

———

Fat Types
General Food Guide

This section presents an <u>Intermediate</u> Food Guide, balanced between the Muscle types (carnivores) and the Thin types (vegetarians). Superimpose the individual type mineral and other information from your type chapter into this Food Guide (which is not for the pargenic type.)

———

Meat/Flesh Intake

Generally, animal protein is acceptable and needed in your diet: red meat should be limited to once weekly or less, while lamb and fish or poultry are excellent in moderation. If this diet is similar to what you are already eating, but you have health problems because of a history of excess acid-ash food intake being so common, then:

- Decrease your carbohydrate and protein intake by about one-third
- Increase your fruit, salad and vegetable intake by about one-third
- Consult with a holistic doctor, preferably one versed in nutritional and emotional evaluation

———

Over-Acid or Over-Alkaline?

Just as a log of wood burned in your fireplace leaves a mineral-ash, food ash refers to the minerals remaining after metabolizing foods in your tissues:

- Fruits and vegetables **alkalinize** tissues
- Proteins and carbohydrates **acidify** tissues

You are usually over-acid due to:

- Accumulated metabolic waste-acids
- Deficient fruit, salad and vegetable intake
- Excessive protein and carbohydrate intake

You need to estimate the ratio of foods you are eating: generally, eat the following *approximate* ratio of foods for your health:

70% *Alkaline-ash* foods (fruits, salads, vegetables)
30% *Acid-ash* foods (complex carbohydrates like starches, grains, cereals, breads, flour products; and proteins)

Approximate your food ratios. On any particular day it does not matter if one meal is mostly alkaline, and another is acid—just try to balance it out for the day! If you make a mistake, forget it and try again tomorrow. It is a subjective call that you make. It is what you do over weeks and months that makes the difference to your health—not on any few days.

The net result is that the Fat types require the plan presented in this chapter for health restoration.

[The following chart shows the fat types, their acid-alkaline reactions, and the percentage of raw foods needed for their healing.]

Fat Types

Acid/Alkaline Genetics

Dietary-Ash and Raw Food Needs

———

This chart shows the Rocine types, their acid or alkaline food needs, and the percentage of raw foods needed for your health and healing.

BODY TYPE	ACID/ALKALINE GENETICS	% DIET ASH	% RAW FOODS
Barotic	Intermediate	50:50	50
Carboferic	Intermediate	50:50	50
Hydripheric	Intermediate	50:50	30
Isogenic	Intermediate	50:50	30
Lipopheric	Intermediate	50:50	50
Oxypheric	Intermediate	50:50	50
Pargenic	Acid	70% alkaline	30

Note that the above percentages will vary depending on aging and the health of individual types.

Notes

- Never eat foods you are allergic to, no matter what I recommend here; if you suspect allergy to a suggested food, eliminate it.
- Minimize your white sugar and alcohol intake.
- Eat the right foods most of the time and the diet will help you; you do not have to live out of a health food store (although such foods are healthier).
- All food lists are in descending order of concentration and value to you as a mineral source; whenever possible, choose foods in the upper half of each list first! One serving is ½ cup.
- If desired, you may interchange lunches for dinners.
- Avoid all junk foods, white sugar, foods with added sugar, and high fructose corn syrup

———

General Food Guide

Breakfasts

EGGS (1-2) with lettuce, tomato, whole grain toast — 1-3 times/week; or

FRUIT SALAD, fresh with citrus fruit and a protein source (low-sugar yogurt, kefir, milk, cottage cheese, cheese, seeds or nuts) — 2-4 times/week; or

COOKED CEREALS, fruit, seeds, whole grain, and nuts — 2-5 times/week; or

OTHER — 0-1 times/week

Eat unlimited fruit, salads, vegetables, with seeds/nuts for snacks. Wheat is a common allergy: avoid white and wheat breads; eat rye, sour dough, or oat breads instead

DAILY LIQUIDS

Pure water — as desired
Fruit and vegetable juices — 0-2 cups
Coffee, caffeine teas — 0-2 cups

[Include selections from your type mineral needs with each meal.]

Lunches

SALADS, mixed green, and 2-4 oz., of protein (fish, poultry, egg, cheese, tofu, seeds or nuts, etc.) [Dressings: use canola or olive oil* and vinegar; or low-fat/calorie dressing] — 2-4 times/week; or

VEGETABLES (steamed) with salad, and yogurt, or cottage cheese (or other breakfast proteins) — 1-2 times/week; or

FRUIT SALAD (see breakfast) — 0-1 times/week

SANDWICH, whole grains with a non-flesh protein (egg, tofu, cheese, etc.) —1-3 times/week; or

POULTRY, FISH, 3-4 oz., with a mixed green salad and/or steamed vegetables (or as a sandwich) —1-2 times/week; or

OTHER — 0-1 times/week

* Other oils less ideal; soybean is common allergen; minimize commercial dressings

[Include selections from your type mineral needs with each meal.]

Dinners

LEAN POULTRY OR FISH *(4-6 oz.)*
— *2-4 times/week*

P.ASTA, PROTEIN *(as above)*
— *1-3 times/week*

VEGETARIAN MEAL *including legumes, tofu,
cheese, cottage cheese, seeds or nuts, egg, etc.*
— *2-4 times/week*

LEAN BEEF *(4-6 oz.) — 0-2 times/*<u>*month*</u>

OTHER — *0-2 times/week*

*Take all of the above with: mixed green salad,
dressing (as before), and/or vegetables (steamed are
best).*

DESSERTS

*Fruits, fresh — as desired
Low-sugar, healthy desserts — 0-3 times/week*

*If you have blood fat problems, cholesterol or
triglycerides, eliminate all beef from your diet, and
see my earlier books.*

*Eat fruit, unlimited salads and vegetables with
seeds/nuts, low-sugar yogurt for snacks.*

**[Include selections from your type mineral
needs with each meal.]**

Fat Types Notes

Do not eat flesh everyday: have it on alternate days only. For munchies, have low calorie items like celery and other vegetables, along with yogurt and cottage cheese, etc. Some of you abuse your beef and red meat intake, perhaps several times weekly—this is a false craving; use your will to combat it if you want to be healthier!

Steamed Vegetables —Minerals are lost in the boiling of vegetables; best is steaming or wok cooking.

Minimize Foods — Only eat them 0-1 times/week! Be sure to eat the recommended foods to help your healing;

Food Combinations —Eating proteins at the same meal with starches often results in indigestion, gas or constipation (along with low blood sugar and making fat). Watch how this inharmonious food combination may be affecting you.

Minimize —
- All fatty foods
- Milk and dairy foods (unless otherwise noted)
- Commercial, sugared, and fatty salad dressings

- Beef, sugar, wines, alcohol, coffee, white sugar, red meats, and processed meats

Vegetarian Proteins — If you choose to be vegetarian, it will help your health after middle-age; because you have semi-carnivorous genes be sure to take a protein supplement of 20-30 grams/day (e.g., soy or egg-white powder in juice).

Healthy Weight — Invariably you hold excessive weight, and in addition to body type factors there may be a medical problem behind your fat storage. By eating according to your body type, you slowly and naturally lose excess weight! Accumulating evidence indicts high-fructose corn syrup as a major cause of increased weight and obesity. Avoid it!

You have a sluggish fat-burning metabolism, and may have an under-active adrenal, thyroid, or pituitary gland resulting in hypoglycemia, and in this instance may need the services of a holistic doctor *(see Appendix* and my earlier books).

In Conclusion

I hope you have enjoyed reading this book. You should now know your body type and have learned some valuable information about how to be a healthier you! Do not forget my previous books on healing yourself.

If you desire further help or information with your body type or health from a holistic viewpoint, email me from page one of my web page: Dr.Stenbeck.net

―――

Appendix

Brief Extracts from
<u>The 22 Unique Body Types</u>

Appendix A

Types
(*Brief extract*)

Type comes from 'typus' meaning an image or impression, the study of types being called typology.

▶ *Rocine: "A combination of mental and structural features is consistently found in people of the same type."*

Rocine wrote that all types are a mixture of positive and negative qualities. He based his work on the biochemical individuality of our *mineral* absorption and utilization. Of course, all minerals are absorbed, but he postulated that different types of people *selectively* absorb certain minerals, to a greater or lesser extent, requiring specific mineral foods for their enhanced health and healing.

▶ *The type information cannot predict what or who you will become, or how successful or not, but your type is capable of bringing a creative excellence to whatever you do in life. If your type has negative qualities that you disagree with, remember that they are only tendencies and may or may not manifest in you.*

This book enlarges on Rocine's premise (early 1900's), integrated with the later research of Herbert Sheldon, M.D., Ph.D., at Harvard University (1930's), along with my fifty years of observations and experience with this subject.

Comparing your shared physical (and sometimes psychological) descriptions with the Celebrity Lists further assists the identification of your type. It is not that you will look exactly like, or be a twin to, any particular celebrity. Look closely at a celebrity's features: face, profile, height, weight, head, etc. If you know something about their talents, beliefs, success and failure spheres, health and weight challenges, attitudes and behaviors, etc., then you get clues as to what your type may be.

———

Understanding Types and Sub-Types

Each of us has a clearly discernible dominant type. Visualize the celebrity examples from movies, politics, sports, the arts and public life, and try to identify with their physical features. Look for similar features, remembering that you will not recognize all attributes in yourself. You are not looking for your twin!

The sub-type issue is the main reason people of the same major type can look so different. Remember that a type description does not characterize you exactly, but depicts your individual variant of a type.

▶ *The type questionnaire pinpoints the major features of that type: if the celebrity examples are unhelpful, you may be an unusual variant (in which case ignore the celebrity issue and give yourself 7 points on Question 1).*

———

Minerals

Minerals are essential life nutrients that accelerate enzyme and chemical reactions and provide a basis for your body typing. Although found in all tissues, different minerals tend to be concentrated in certain organs, their presence or absence contributing to the healing of such tissues; e.g., zinc accelerates prostate healing; calcium and manganese promote bone, joint and connective tissue healing.

Specific foods nurture each type, some people needing meats for their health others needing a vegetarian diet. A high potassium diet nurtures one person, while another needs high sulfur, calcium, zinc, or another mineral.

Mineral Digestion and Absorption

Compared to vitamins, minerals are *difficult* to digest, absorb, and utilize. In people with strong digestive systems, this aspect may not be important. The following factors should be in place for optimal mineral metabolism:

1. Stomach Hydrochloric Acid Production
2. Parathyroid Hormone Balance
3. Organ Toxic Metal and Chemical Removal
   [See details in <u>The 22 Unique Body Types</u>.]

———

Total Body Healing

Note that from a holistic healing perspective, in addition to minerals and type information, the following healing factors are necessary:

> *Nutrient Balance*
> *Mental Balance*
> *Emotional Balance*
> *Spiritual Balance*
> *Detoxifying Integrity*

The above factors are all important to your total healing especially if you are interested in self-healing (see my earlier books).

———

Appendix B

Researchers
(Brief extract)

The predominant workers in this area of human individuality from around 1880's to the 1960's are Herbert Sheldon, M.D., Ph.D., Roger Williams, Ph.D., and Victor Rocine, D.Sc.

Much information on Sheldon's research exists on-line and in medical psychology libraries; for interested readers there are other lines of research published in the last century. This present book is primarily about Rocine's body types.

Herbert Sheldon M.D., Ph.D.

In contrast to Rocine, Sheldon at Harvard University in the 1930's was trained in the scientific method and did painstaking research and publishing on human individuality. In comparing his findings with Rocine's work, a direct putative correlation is visible.

Roger J. Williams, Ph.D.

Another significant researcher in human individuality is the renowned scientist and biochemist, Roger J. Williams. He demonstrated that different people have varying levels of nutrients, enzymes, and other metabolic chemicals in their bloodstreams.

▶ *Williams's research firmly expands on the premise of individual nutritional needs in human beings. If interested in his research, I highly recommend his book Biochemial Individuality.*

Victor Rocine, D.Sc.

Note that when a negative feature is indicated, say neurotic tendencies, all members of the type are <u>not</u> that way; it is a type tendency reported by Rocine.

Rocine studied type-related diseases finding links between mineral and dietary factors with individual types and their diseases. In each body type, one or more dominant minerals are preferentially absorbed and utilized over other minerals.

He recognized discrete body types from their physical appearance finding genetically based mineral dominance to be the determining feature. He also correlated their physical features with psychological characteristics.

———

Appendix C

Genetics, Types, and Diet
(Brief extract)

This section deals with how nervous system genetics helps determine your eating choices for health: you are either born to be a predominant meat eater, a partial or complete vegetarian, or something between the two. The genetic factor determining this dietary aspect is the *sympathetic and parasympathetic* components of your central nervous system. This represents a basic factor in eating for health.

This chapter helps you understand your dietary inheritance, although instinctively, you may already have arrived there!

- If born **sympathetic** dominant you are *genetically acid*, desiring a predominantly *vegetarian* diet for your health (about 70% fruit, salad, vegetables to 30% proteins and carbohydrates).

- If born **parasympathetic** dominant you are *genetically alkaline*, desiring a predominantly *carnivorous* diet for your health (about 70% proteins, carbohydrates to 30% fruits, salads, vegetables). Few of you ever choose to become vegetarian because of the difficulty in satisfying your protein needs without meats.

- If born ***intermediate*** dominant you may eat food groups with little concern for the acid/alkaline factor. However, after age 40, you need a semi-vegetarian diet for healthy eating.

Chart of Relative Nervous System Dominance

In the following Chart, if you relate to many of the symptoms on one side you probably have that nervous system dominance; relating to both sides indicates *Intermediate* dominance.

If Vegetarian (Over-acid) --
Eat 70% fruits, salads, vegetables
And 30% proteins, carbohydrates

If Carnivore (Over-alkaline) --
Eat 70% proteins, carbohydrates
And 30% fruits, salads, vegetables

If Intermediate --
Eat 50:50 of acid and alkaline-ash foods

Make an *approximate* estimate of your daily acid and alkaline food intake (such ratios varying from type to type).

Symptoms of Relative Genetic Dominance

Vegetarians (Over-acid)	*Carnivores* (Over-alkaline)
Sympathetic Dominance	*Parasympathetic Dominance*
little or no flesh desire	desire flesh
easily constipated	rarely constipated
slow digestion	fast digestion
easily dehydrated	not dehydrated
strong thirst	low thirst
pale face	flushed face
high pulse after food	slow pulse after food
easy gag reflex	slow gag reflex
cool dry skin	moist warm skin
nervous stomach	calm stomach
little eyelid blinking	much blinking
nervous tendency	mostly calm
slower healing	faster healing
low oxygen-uptake	good oxygen-uptake
easily breathless	seldom breathless
insomnia common	sleep easier
few muscle cramps	some night cramps
calcium deposits rare	get calcium deposits

Appendix D

Help Identifying your Body Type with Dr. Stenbeck

If you desire help in identifying your body type, follow these instructions, and answer the questionnaire. For further information and fees, send me an email from page one of the website:

DrStenbeck.net

First name: _____

Country of birth: _____

Upload photos and send to the above website:

■ Head and shoulders: front and side views

■ Full body: front and side views

■ Also 1-2 teenage views

■ If possible, casual photos of mother, father, siblings

MY TYPE CLASS MAY BE: _____

   (Thin, Muscle, or Fat)

AGE   -   _____

HEIGHT   -   _____ feet/inches

MY WEIGHT -   _____ pounds

   Heaviest at age: _____

- Lightest as adult: _____

- Estimate age 15: _____

VISION - Excellent Average   Poor:

HAIR -   Natural color: _____

- Thin/thick?   _____

- balding?   _____

SKIN - Quality: _____

- History of acne, boils, other:

_____

_____

TEETH   - Strong   Weak   Dentures

- Cavity history: Many   Moderate Few

MUSCLES - Strong   Average   Weak

Sports played _____

JOINTS   - Strong   Average   Weak

HEALTH - Childhood diseases?

_____

_____

- Adult diseases?

_____

AVERAGE DIET

- Beef _____ (times/week)

 - Poultry _____ (times/week)

 - Fish _____ (times/week)

 - Eggs _____ (times/week)

 - Water _____ (glasses/day):

- Vegetarian? Vegan? _____

- Other? _____

 - Did your childhood diet differ? _____

The above will help me know who you are! I will send you a follow-up questionnaire for further help in identifying your body type.

Appendix E

On-line Health Consultation with Dr. Stenbeck

For further information, or to comment on this book, or to receive a response on any health issue from a holistic viewpoint, send an email inquiry from page one of my website:

DrStenbeck.net

Following that, I will suggest further healing needs, which we may pursue with an on-line consult.

———

Appendix F

Notes

See my book <u>*The 22 Unique Body Types,*</u> available at the usual online source, for further information and details on all of the 22 Types. The Appendix in that book has further information about:

Mineral Functions and Food Sources

Further Reading

———